# Contents

# Alfalfa

Alfalfa, which is a perennial herb, has a long list of dietary and medicinal uses and research has proven that Alfalfa might lower blood levels of cholesterol and glucose. It is also helpful in diabetes control. Many take Alfalfa supplements orally and is has been proven safe except in a small percentage of people where it produces lupus like symptoms. In the seeds and sprouts of Alfalfa, amino acid L-canavanine is present and that is what is thought to cause this reaction. However, this is not present in the leaves of the Alfalfa. The whole leaf and the herb are what are rendered from the Alfalfa plant.

Since the sixth century the Chinese have used Alfalfa to relieve fluid retention and swelling. The Arabs were the first to find Alfalfa and they named it "the father of all foods." The leaves of the Alfalfa plant are very rich in minerals and nutrients, including potassium, calcium, magnesium, and carotene. The Arabs first fed it to their horses because they believed the Alfalfa made them swift and mighty. Alfalfa has been an animal crop for over a thousand years but is also used as an herbal medicine.

Alfalfa is a good diuretic and also a good laxative. It also works well for urinary tract infections, and kidney, bladder and prostrate disorders. The latest and greatest discovery of Alfalfa is the benefits that it might provide for lowering cholesterol because there are certain agents in Alfalfa that stick to cholesterol which keeps it from remaining in the blood stream. Further, it may also have a very strong relationship with lowering blood sugar levels.

When it comes to Alfalfa it is something that many people enjoy in their cuisine. It is good in salads and some people eat it as a vegetable all alone. Many people claim that eating Alfalfa is a big part of eating healthy. Besides wheat grass and algae, Alfalfa has the most nutritional value. It is high in fiber, vitamins, minerals, and has all of the required digestive enzymes. Juice of Alfalfa is rich in elements which are useful for the growth of hair and the prevention of hair loss. The juice of alfalfa along with carrot and lettuce juice, taken daily, promote hair growth to a remarkable extent.

Alfalfa is also great for reducing fevers and is very good for the blood. It contains natural fluoride and prevents tooth decay. Alfalfa also takes out minor diseases like Whooping Cough. It makes a great tea because when the Alfalfa leaves steep in the hot water it is a source of nitrogen. The tea is not only made for human consumption because people who grow Irises and Delphiniums just love Alfalfa tea because of the great effect that it has on the plants when used as a foliar spray. Many with a green thumb also use Alfalfa as mulch for their flower beds.

It is warned by avid Alfalfa lovers that you likely will not like the way that it tastes in your mouth, it may feel like it is burning the tip of your tongue and you actually might just completely dislike it however, they urge you to not give up because it is an acquired taste and you will begin to like it. The best news is that soon after eating it regularly you will find that your appetite for heavier foods will diminish.

As a matter of fact, Alfalfa has some drawbacks at some situations like it is not recommended to use as contraceptive and canavinine as it reactivates lupus erythematous and reversible pancytopenia, therefore it should be avoided if you ever suffered from this disease. It should also be avoided in pregnancy and during medication for thinning of blood and anticoagulant. Too much intake may damage red blood cells and cause photosentivity.

# Asafoetida

Asafoetida has been also referred to as the "Food of the Gods." The main part of this plant that is used is the resin which makes up a volatile oil. The history of this herb is amazing as it was used frequently back in time by Alexander the Great for flavoring. That was back in 4 B.C. still in early times, Asafoetida was used to treat gas and the bloating associated with it. Carrying through time the resin gum is used often for vegetarian dishes that are prepared in India. Today, it is one of the main flavorings in Worcestershire sauce.

Asafoetida is an herbal plant that has many diverse uses such as an aid for digestion, a remedy for headaches, an antidote, and an expectorant. Asafoetida has been known to be used on some mental impairment but not very often has it been shown to make any significant difference except for mild anxiety. Therefore it focuses primarily on bodily functions where it can do greater good. Asafoetida might help against high blood levels due to fats, cholesterols and triglycerides.

As mentioned earlier, it works on gas and the bloating associated with it but further it also eases indigestion, rids stomach cramps, and helps with constipation, which is Asafoetida's contribution in the digestion department. When it comes to headaches, when Asafoetida is mixed with water it is showing great promise for the treatment of migraines and tension headaches. As an antidote, it works great for snake bites and an insect repellant when it is mixed with garlic.

As an expectorant the Asafoetida oil helps to rid the body of excess mucus and eases the respiratory system. Many use it for whooping cough, asthma, and bronchitis. Where expectoration is a problem asafetida helps in expelling accumulated cough. Some mixtures that seem to blend together well for coughs and as expectorants are roasted fresh resinous gum powder with real ghee or a mixture of asafetida powder with honey, white onion juice, betel nut juice and dry ginger.

Asafoetida has a very unpleasant odor, so bad that many call it the "Devil's Dung." The foul odor comes from the resin that is removed from the plant's stem and root. Asafoetida is a species of the fennel plant but a relative to the carrot. The wicked odor is formed from the organic sulfur

4

compound found as part of the essential oils. When it comes to the value of the Asafoetida tree, the older, the better and trees less than four years of age are virtually worthless.

When buying Asafoetida in the marketplace it will likely be available in three different forms, one is called tears which are commonly sold in Chinese pharmacies and characteristically may have fragments of root and earth. It is also sold in a paste which is very commonly used as a condiment for flavoring such dishes as curry, to flavor beans, sauces, pickles, and many use it as a substitute for garlic. Coumarins chemicals are present in Asafoetida that can thin the blood.

In case of children, Asafoetida is helpful in the disorders of nervous system. When mixed with oil, massaging on neck can prevent several children diseases. For women, Asafoetida is beneficial in problems such as sterility, leucorrhoea, difficult and painful menstruation, premature labor, unwanted abortion and sterility. After childbirth, Asafoetida is prescribed Asafoetida is also prescribed to women after childbirth because it helps in digestion in women.

A few other unique things that Asafoetida is used for is that if used in recipes regularly it has been suggested that it may increase the chances of male fertility. Often it is used for toothaches as well. According to modern research, Asafoetida is helpful in swine flu.

# Balsam of Tolu

Balsam of Tolu is an herb that comes from a very tall tree that can be found in Columbia, Peru, Venezuela, Argentina, Brazil, Paraguay, and Bolivia. This herbal plant has also been called Balsam of Peru because it was originally exported primarily from Peru but that is no longer the case. The resin of this tree is what is most valuable and is retrieved in the same fashion that one collects the valuable properties from a rubber tree by tapping into it. The gummy resin that comes from the tree is then turned into balsam. Today, the main exporters of Balsam of Tolu are El Salvador, Columbia, and Venezuela.

In earlier times it was tribal groups from Mexico and Central America that used the leaves of Balsam of Tolu to treat such common ailments as external wounds, asthma, colds, flu, and arthritis. Some native Indians used the bark in a powered form as an underarm deodorant while others found it best for lung and cold ailments. Those who originated in the rainforest tribes used Balsam of Tolu quite frequently for many medicinal purposes such as abscesses, asthma, bronchitis, catarrh, headache, rheumatism, sores, sprains, tuberculosis, venereal diseases, and wounds. It contains ingredients that help break up congestion.

As this herbal plant grew in popularity, it was the Europeans who wanted in on the action and soon the Germans were using it for pharmaceutical purposes as well. They found that Balsam of Tolu worked very well for antibacterial, antifungal, and antiphrastic purposes so they immediately started using it for such things as scabies, ringworm, lice, minor ulcerations, wounds, bedsores, and diaper rash. Today, it is used very often in topical salves for the treatment of wounds, ulcers, and scabies.

It can be found in hair tonics, antidandruff shampoos, feminine hygiene sprays and as a natural fragrance in soaps, detergents, creams, lotions, and perfumes. In the early 1800's, the United States wanted to utilize Balsam of Tolu as well but used it mainly for treatments as cough suppressants and respiratory aids used in cough lozenges and syrups, for sore throats, and as a vapor inhalant for respiratory distress. It is also inhaled by some people to treat hoarseness and croup.

Balsam of Tolu has a vanilla like smell and taste and it is used mostly for flavoring cough syrups, soft drinks, confectionaries, and chewing gums. Balsam of Tolu is widely available now in the U.S. The essential oil distilled from the gum is sold in small bottles and used topically, in aromatherapy. The fragrance is considered to be healing and comforting. It is useful for meditation and relaxation which is why it has become so popular amongst the world of aromatherapy. Balsam of Tolu has a very unique aroma which makes it excellent for exotic floral fragrances.

Generally its topical use is recommended for skin rashes, eczema, and skin parasites such as scabies, ringworm, and head lice. Balsam of Tolu is considered sensitizing oil which means that it is more likely to cause an allergic reaction to the skin or be a skin irritant than other herbal oils might be in people who are sensitive or commonly have allergies to plants and herbs.

# Basil

Originally, Basil was not the most popular herb in the bunch. Actually there were some who simply hated it, mainly the ancient people. The name basil means "be fragrant" but still various cultures battled with a love hate relationship over basil. Americans and Romans loved it while Hindus plant it in their homes as a sign of happiness. On the contrary it was the Greeks who despised it most but those from India and Persia were not too fond of it either. One place that took a special liking to Basil was Italy and to this day not many people prepare a classic pasta sauce without the Basil.

To this day basil and tomato sauce have formed somewhat of a marriage almost globally. Basil is very easy to grow as long as the temperature does not fall below 50 degrees and is in full sunshine. It is popularly used both in the fresh form as well as the dried. A rare known fact about Basil is that the longer it simmers in a dish the more the flavor intensifies. This makes sense as to why people simmer their pasta sauces for so long, to bring out all of the rich herb flavors. Normally in pasta sauces Basil is used in combination with Oregano. However, Basil is not just used for pasta or tomato sauce, it is also used for flavoring fish, vegetables, meats, and soups.

If you decide to grow an herb garden, you can thank the Basil plants for keeping the flies away as flies are also part of the group that does not care for Basil. Another interesting fact about Basil is that it was considered a royal herb with a strong association pertaining to love. Basil had a relationship with how men of a much earlier time planned on proposing to their fair maidens. The man would bring a branch of Basil and if the woman accepted his gift she silently agreed to love him and be faithful to him for eternity.

Basil is related to the Mint family and just knowing that should give you a good idea that it will have many medicinal uses as well. Right away most people associate anything mint with aiding the digestive system and also for its anti-gas properties. Herbalists use Basil quite commonly for health ailments such as stomach cramps, vomiting, constipation, headaches and anxiety. When Basil is used for these purposes it is generally made into a hot tea for drinking. Some also claim that a nice hot cup of Basil tea can contribute greatly to a good night's sleep. At herbal stores you can also purchase Basil capsules as well if you do not care for the taste of the tea.

Basil is used to treat respiratory and chest problems. It helps to get rid of cold and flu symptoms. Basil has anti-bacterial effects and retards the production of bacteria. Basil has strengthening effect on the kidney. In case of renal stone the juice of basil leaves and honey, if taken regularly for 6 months it will expel them via the urinary tract. Basil leaves are very useful for mouth infections and used for the treatment of ulcers. Its leaves are usually dried and used for brushing purposes. Regular use of Basil herb can prevent heart failure.

Basil is still one of the most common household herbs used today and in most areas of culinary art it is a necessity there too. When used in its freshest form, Basil is torn from the plant and then just minced up with a knife. Usually somewhere nearby the Basil you will find some olive oil, garlic, and someone getting ready to prepare a fantastic tomato sauce.

# Chapter 5 - Belladonna

Belladonna is not an herb that you are going to want to stock your pantry with. While it has its benefits, this is an herb that can be very dangerous and sometimes even fatal. It has some medicinal properties to it and has an interesting history but it can be very dangerous. The nickname "deadly nightshade" is a good clue of its potency. There is however a tincture that comes from this plant that is used for medicinal purposes. Belladonna is a perennial herb that is native to Europe and Asia Minor but is now grown quite often in the United States, Europe, and India. When the plant is in full bloom the plant is harvested and then dried for use.

The most important contribution from Belladonna is atropine which is an important agent that is useful in dilating the pupils of the eye. This has proven to be very beneficial. Even small doses of atropine can cause the heart rate to increase. Some cough syrups are known to contain atropine and are used for bronchitis and whooping cough. Further it is used to soothe the stomach lining prior to an anesthetic being administered and also for peptic ulcers.

Belladonna goes by many different names but has been used for over 500 years. While growing in the wild, which belladonna commonly does, a slight dose can be fatal. In the earliest times when Belladonna was first used it was cosmetic purposes. Women felt that if they used it to dilate their pupils that they would look more sexy and alluring. That is why the name Belladonna means "beautiful lady" in Italian. Yet, it is still used in many eye doctors' offices across the country to this day.

Belladonna also has other great benefits for purposes of what it is used for today as it has the ability to dry up bodily fluids such as breast milk, saliva, perspiration, and mucous. The alkaloids in Belladonna are used for many conditions such as gastrointestinal disorders such as colitis, diverticulitis, irritable bowel syndrome, colic, diarrhea, and peptic ulcer. It also works for asthma, excessive sweating, excessive nighttime urination and incontinence, headaches and migraines, muscle pains and spasms, motion sickness, Parkinson's disease, and biliary colic.

Quite often Belladonna is used as homeopathic remedies such as the common cold, earaches, fever, menstrual cramps, sunstroke, toothaches, headaches, sore throats, and boils. How the patient ingests and how much they ingest is determined by a few various factors such as their symptoms, mood, and overall temperament. When Belladonna is administered for homeopathic use it is highly diluted because of the toxicity level of it.

No one should ever use Belladonna as a self-help measure and it should only be taken under the care of a qualified doctor. The doses given of Belladonna are always in very low doses. When Belladonna is prescribed it is either added to sugar pellets or mixed with other types of drugs and is available by prescription only. So while it is clear that Belladonna is an extremely dangerous herb it is also very beneficial when used correctly.

# Burdock

Burdock is a plant that is related to the daisy family. It is also closely related to Echinacea, Dandelion, and Feverfew. Burdock is an herb but it is one that has been much neglected when it comes to getting attention. Back in ancient times the Greeks used the roots, the seeds, and the greens and used them for healing purposes. Throughout the Middle Ages Burdock was used for both food and medicine.

The Native Americans knew Burdock very well. They used the whole plant as food. Indians also used Burdock to treat rheumatism. In ancient times, it was used to purify the blood and aid circulation. Some tribes honored its curing powers.

Burdock is usually found in the United States, Europe, Japan and China. Burdock contains many vitamins, minerals, fiber, essential oils and phytosterols due to which it has high usage in medicines.

Traditionally, seeds of the burdock are crushed to make a mixture that provided relief for measles, arthritis, tonsillitis, throat pain, and viruses like the common cold. Today, Burdock is still used for such things as easing liver problems and digestive disorders. It was also found to be very effective for cleansing the skin for problems such as acne and also to assist in digestive problems. To this day throughout Europe the stalk and the greens are still eaten because they hold such valuable nutrition and vitamin values.

As more and more research is being done on Burdock many new and interesting discoveries are cropping up. A relationship is being examined between Burdock and its anti-fungal and anti-bacterial properties, and even more important it is showing signs of possibly being able to fight against tumors and could be a cancer fighting agent as well. Research has shown that since many of the cancer causing compounds are in almost all foods which are then eaten and stored in the human fat tissues that Burdock might very well be of help in fighting cancer because of the role that it can play in depleting these mutagens.

Burdock is also very helpful in strengthening the immune system when it has become weakened by environmental factors. When mixed with other herbs such as Dandelion and Ginger it can be a very powerful blood purifier. The most unique fact about Burdock is that it has a very high amount of insulin which is a natural occurring chemical within the body that mimics actions of insulin. Because of this, Burdock has been successful in helping combat hypoglycemia and pre diabetes conditions.

If you look for Burdock in the market you may find it called Gobo instead as that is what some refer to it as. It is often combined with other vegetables or added to Tofu. Some boil Burdock while others sauté or deep fry it. Many have said it might not be such a good idea to look at Burdock before you eat it because you might change your mind about taking a bite.

It looks thick, dark, and woody but indeed the opposite is true when it comes to the taste. Burdock is well recognized as a health food because it has low calorie content and a high fiber intake. It is also loaded with potassium, iron, and calcium. People claim that Burdock tastes like nothing else. In other words it has a taste all of its own.

The best description that people can agree on when it comes to the flavor of Burdock is that it is sweet yet earthy, with a tender and crisp texture. It is often added to stews, soups, and stir fries. In the form of food, Burdock is highly nutritional and full of vitamins but in retrospect Burdock is also an effective herb for bringing the body back into balance. Burdock has a side effect that it can make worse the skin conditions before healing.

# Catnip

"Catnip" is the common name for a perennial herb of the mint family. Catnip is native to Europe and is imported into the United States. In North America it is a common widespread weed. Catnip is most popular with cats and the reaction that it causes in them when they receive some dried nip from their owner. They roll around in it in all of their glory. The fact is that humans do not smell what cats smell when it comes to catnip so humans do not react the same way that cats do. It is known that the chemical nepetalactone in catnip is the thing that triggers the response. Apparently, it somehow kicks off a stereotypical pattern in cats that are sensitive to the chemical.

Catnip can be grown indoors. It only require a window with six hour daylight. Just make sure to keep it moist at all times, and pinch off flowers to encourage leaf growth. Catnip requires most soil. Ph level of soil should in the range of 6.1 to 7.8.

In humans catnip has been used for several ailments including the treatment of colic, headache, toothache, colds, and spasms. It is also known to induce sleep in most people but it others it can have a counter effect. Catnip also has antibacterial properties to it too. In the 15th century the English cooks would season meats with catnip and also add a pinch to salads. Many people also prefer catnip tea to Chinese tea. Some of the agents in catnip also act as a very effective cockroach repellent. It has actually been proven to be more effective by 100% than DEET.

When taken orally, catnip shows a great benefit for anxiety, insomnia, and nervousness. Nepetalactone is the active ingredient in catnip and is commonly used as an herbal sedative. Because of this it is also great for easing migraine headaches, stomach complaints, and also reduces swelling associated with arthritis, hemorrhoids, and soft tissue injuries. Catnip can be purchased in a liquid, dried, or a capsule form. It is the dried form that is commonly brewed into a tea. Folklore has it that if catnip is smoked it might produce minor hallucinogenic effects but that has since been disregarded. It was also said that when children would throw fits that catnip would be able to calm them and also stop children from having nightmares.

Some claims have been made that catnip is a distant relative of marijuana. There really is no validity to this claim except for the way that the cats act when they roll around in the nip which looks like they have a buzz. When the cat rolls around in it a euphoric effect is displayed but if the cat eats any of the nips, he is certain to fall fast asleep. Catnip has been called the mysterious herb by many. It is related to common kitchen herbs like thyme and sage, and can be easily cultivated as a houseplant.

Another fact about Catnip is that as much as cats seem to love it is as much as mosquitoes hate it. These are all the things that make catnip such a unique herb that it has the ability to entertain cats, it has medicinal properties, there are a few funny myths about it and is an insect repellant all in one.

Catnip has not any side effects. But pregnant women should avoid its use as it can cause uterine contraction. This herb has also shown no contraindications with other medicines. According to some people, Catnip smells like skunk.

# Chamomile

Chamomile is an herb that has been used for thousands of years for many ailments including gas, diarrhea, stomach upset, sleeplessness, and anxiety. It can also be used topically for certain skin lesions. The Chamomile plant has flowering tops and these are what are used for making tea and other herbal remedies that include Chamomile.

Harvesting Chamomile is a delicate process as its seeds need light to germinate. Best time for its growth is August. Otherwise, they can be started indoors in propagation flats in March and transplanted outdoors after a hardening off period. In most cases, direct planting in the garden after all chance of frost has passed are successful, as well. Chamomile is very resistant after firm growth.

When Chamomile tops are stewed and then drained the liquid is a deep yellow color and can be lightly sweetened if preferred. It has a very unique taste to it and many women used to make sure they always had a few baby bottles tucked safely away in the refrigerator in case their baby got gas. It was used before the days of over the counter gas relief drops and although there is no scientific validity to it, it always seemed to make the baby stop wailing and fall fast asleep.

Chamomile produces an oil that when isolated turns a very unique bluish color and this has very distinct anti-inflammatory properties to it so it has been known to work very well on skin infections, eczema, and inflamed skin. This would be Chamomile in its topical form rather than the flowers or the tea from the flowers. Again, remember that Chamomile was around for a long time before many over the counter and prescription medications were so readily available. For years all many people had to rely on was herbal remedies that were likely passed down from generations and possibly continued to be passed down even after the newer medications did come to the forefront. It was also given to women for menstrual cramps in the days before Midol and Pamprin.

Chamomile is anti-inflammatory and anti-spasmodic. It calms process of inflammation both inside and outside of the body. Chamomile acts to sooth the smooth muscles lining the digestive tract, relieving irritable symptoms. Outside the body, it is used to treat mild burns, including sunburn, rashes, sores and even eye inflammation. As an anti-spasmodic, Chamomile has the power to relax muscles and nerves. It is used commonly to treat anxiety disorders and insomnia, muscle pain and muscle strains. Chamomile has certain active compounds which are helpful in anti-anxiety medications, which promote relaxation in the brain and nervous system.

Often when small children had bug bites, diaper rashes, or eczema, the mother would fill a stocking with Chamomile and oatmeal and let it soak in the tub with her children. It was very effective in stopping the itch and improving the diaper rash. Chamomile was also used in combination with other herbs for a lot of other purposes such as if one felt nauseous, a combination of Chamomile, shredded licorice root, fennel seeds, and peppermint would cure that pretty quickly. Because Chamomile is part of the Ragweed family you should not ingest it if you have an allergy to Ragweed.

Some people love to sip a hot cup of Chamomile tea with no ailments at all, just because they enjoy it. Pregnant and nursing mothers are advised to stay away from all herbs but Chamomile is the exception to this rule. It is completely safe for anyone to drink at any time. It has even been known to help teething babies too. On a final note Chamomile has been known to be an excellent hair conditioner and to sooth scalps. When mixed with a bit of lemon and sunshine it has also been known to give subtle natural highlights to hair.

# Cilantro

Cilantro is a very fast growing herb which can be grown just about anywhere. It is a relative of the carrot family and is sometimes called Chinese parsley and Coriander. Cilantro actually is the leaves and stems of the Coriander plant.

It has a very strong unique odor and is relied on heavily for Mexican, Asian, and Caribbean cuisine. Cilantro also resembles Parsley which is not surprising since the two are related. For thousands of years Cilantro has been around, first in Egypt, India, and China and then it was introduced to Mexico and Peru where it is still used with chilies when making masterful food dishes. It has since become very popular in certain parts of the United States as well. Today, Cilantro has lost its popularity in Europe as most Europeans are repulsed by the very smell of it.

Cilantro is a Greek word that means "koris" which in English means bedbug oddly enough because it is said by many that Cilantro smells like a bedbug. The Chinese did not seem to mind because they add Cilantro to their various love potions because to them it symbolizes immortality and has aphrodisiac properties to it. Many also say that it is an appetite stimulant. Cilantro is very easy to find in pretty much any local grocery store or fruit market any time of the year.

Cilantro has an interesting history to it and has showed up many times throughout history. Keep in mind that Cilantro is also in part Coriander, and some seeds were found in King Tut's tomb. It is also mentioned in the Old Testament and was used by physicians dated back as far as Hippocrates. The Ancient Egyptians used Cilantro for such things as headaches and urinary tract infections.

Cilantro can also mask the scent of rotting meat and it was used for that purpose quite frequently by earlier cultures. It would be fair to say that Cilantro is an herbal plant that has two identities since Cilantro is what the plant is referred to in its earliest stages and when it is fully developed it then becomes Coriander. Cilantro grows very quickly but also dies very quickly but it can easy grow in a pot on your windowsill. It is always best to harvest Cilantro before it bolts or blooms. If you wait too long to harvest Cilantro what will happen is that you will be harvesting Coriander because it will then be all seed.

Today, Cilantro can be found just about anywhere in the United States and is a garnish on almost every plate served in an upscale restaurant. The odd thing about Cilantro is that most people either love it or they hate it, usually there is no in between.

Cilantro has an anti-bacterial action against many bacteria like Salmonella. It is a natural treatment for chelation treatment. Cilantro is helpful in case of nausea. It helps in digestion and relieves intestinal gas. Blood sugar and cholesterol levels are also lowered by using Cilantro. It is also a source of healthy ingredients like, iron, magnesium and fibers. Cilantro has antioxidant properties and also reduces minor swellings. It has immune boosting property. In case of diarrhea, Cilantro has fruitful effects.

As a medicinal herb, coriander is usually considered safe. Because of the volatile found in the seeds, coriander may cause allergic reaction and some people may experience dermatitis after handling the leaves. Breastfeeding and pregnant women should not use excessive amount of this herb.

# Cloves

Cloves are definitely one of the most distinct herbs around but ironically enough, cloves have been around forever and are not finished doing business just yet. Usually if you cannot get your hands on some cloves, Allspice can be a substitute. Cloves have some preservative properties to them but they work well as an antiseptic, expectorant, anesthetic, or an emmenogogue, working well on the kidneys, the spleen and the stomach.

Some make a combination of cloves, bay leaves, cinnamon, and marjoram for a hot tea that helps bronchitis, asthma, coughs, a tendency to infection, tuberculosis, altitude sickness, nervous stomach, nausea, diarrhea, flatulence, indigestion, dyspepsia, gastroenteritis, the side effects of lobelia, and depression. Sometimes people mix cloves with hot water, again making a tea and claim that it helps them get a good night's sleep.

Cloves and ginger is a sure way to settle the stomach and stop vomiting. If you combine equal parts of cloves and basil it is supposed to detox meals from the body. Cloves have been used for failing eyesight and tooth problems. It was used for earaches very often throughout history as putting a little warmed oil of clove on a piece of cotton and in your ear was certain to rid any earache. Mostly, cloves are known for being warm and spicy but also have a strong relationship with pain relief, easing nausea and vomiting, and improving digestion. Cloves also kill intestinal parasites and act as an antimicrobial agent against fungi and bacteria. It has also been suggested that cloves have antihistamine properties as well.

Do not be too quick to pass off the possibilities of cloves and aromatherapy as the two have a very strong bond between them. Since cloves have such a positive and stimulating effect on the mind they pair up great with other oils for aromatherapy purposes. In the 16th and 17th centuries cloves were worth their weight in gold however it is the clove oil that is most essential. In Indonesia many people smoke clove cigarettes and that did spill over into the United States for a while but lost most of its vigor when it was found that clove cigarettes could cause adult respiratory distress syndrome.

The word clove comes from the Latin word "clavus" which means nail. If you have ever looked at a clove you will notice that it does resemble a nail. Many people use whole cloves when they cook ham by sticking the spiky part around the outer edges of the ham for extra flavor. Indian curries cannot do without cloves but it is also used in pickles, sauces, Worcestershire sauce, and even spice cakes that are baked from scratch.

Clove is used extensively in dental care for relieving toothache, sore gums and oral ulcers. Clove oil reduces infections, wounds, insect bites and stings. Clove has an excellent aiding property for skin disorders, such as acne. It is also used as a blood purifier and useful in case of premature ejaculation. Clove has anti-fungal properties and also used for cancer prevention.

Throughout history cloves has never been forgotten but has lost some of its popularity. Some still use it as a spice and some for minor dentistry and even still more for the purpose of aromatherapy. People still look at cloves as an "old fashioned" herb. For some families it has been passed down through generations and in the pantry still sits a jar of whole cloves for that special ham dinner.

# Dandelion

The Dandelion is an herbaceous plant that really is much more than just a nuisance in your yard. For all purposes, the Dandelion leaves are at their best just as they emerge from the ground and they are very distinct as nothing really resembles this at all. Depending on when you harvest the Dandelion leaves will determine the bitterness of them but it is an appealing bitterness.

These leaves that are considered an herb blend nicely with salads and do well either sautéed or steamed. Many claim the taste is similar to that of endive. People who are into eating the fruits of nature claim that it is perfectly acceptable to eat the Dandelion flower as well. Some claim that they make outstanding fritters if they are battered up and fried and make a colorful contribution to any stir fry.

Dandelion leaves are actually extremely nutritious, much more so than any herb that can be purchased in the stores. They are higher in beta carotene than carrots are and they have more iron and calcium than spinach does. Dandelion leaves are also full of vitamins B-1, B-2, B-5, B-6, B-12, C, E, P, D, biotin, inositol, potassium, phosphorus, magnesium, and zinc. Dandelion root is one of the safest and most popular herbal remedies on the market and is widely used today.

Traditionally it can be made into a tonic that is known for strengthening the entire body, especially the liver and gallbladder because it promotes the flow of bile. Dandelion root contains taraxacin so it reduces the inflammation to the bile ducts and reduces gallstones. It is commonly used for Hepatitis, liver swelling, and jaundice. It also helps with indigestion.

Dandelion Leaf also serves to protect the liver from damage. Many people use the herb to rinse out their liver after drinking excess amounts of alcohol or after eating unhealthful foods. In fact, if you are taking prescription drugs such as antibiotics, Dandelion Leaf may flush them out of your bloodstream at a faster than normal rate. Therefore, you should be aware of any potential conflicts between this herbal ingredient and medications.

This plant also goes by the French name, Pissenlit. Ironically enough when used in the tea form made by the leaves or the root has a tendency to act as a diuretic on the kidneys. Over the counter diuretics have a tendency to suck the potassium out of the body but not the Dandelion leaves. Dandelion root tea has helped some actually avoid surgery for urinary stones. Dandelions are really just good for overall health and well-being so just about anyone could benefit from a cup of dandelion tea. Many herbalists say that incorporated the Dandelion plant into dinner each night will assist in easier digestion.

When you take a Dandelion plant and break the stem you will find a milky white substance inside. This substance is great for removing warts, pimples, moles, calluses, soothing of bee stings, and blisters. Some other things that Dandelion has been popular in the past for is making Dandelion jam and others use it for a coffee substitute when it is roasted and ground Dandelion root. Many also drink Dandelion wine.

Today, Europeans use plenty of Dandelion roots to make herbal medicines and find it hard to believe that Americans refer to this highly beneficial plant as a weed when it has such positive benefits for the liver, spleen, kidneys, bladder, and the stomach.

Dandelion is generally safer to use. It can cause allergic reactions to some people. People with an allergy to ragweed, chrysanthemums, marigold, chamomile, yarrow, daisies or iodine, may need to avoid dandelion. In case of bile ducks blockage, Dandelion should be avoided. Dandelion can cause overproduction of stomach acids; therefore those who are affected by long term and persistent cases of stomach ulcer or gastritis should take extreme caution before using dandelion. Dandelion is a diuretic and may increase the excretion of drugs from the body.

# Echinacea

Echinacea was used frequently by Native American Tribes for a wide variety of conditions. At least 14 tribes used Echinacea for ailments such as coughs, colds, sore throats, and infections. In 1887, Echinacea was introduced into U.S. medical practice, and it grew in popularity. By the early twentieth century Echinacea had become the top selling herb in America. However, with the discovery of penicillin and other "wonder drugs," the popularity of Echinacea eventually diminished. Even though it continued to be used in America it fell completely into disuse in the 1930's after it was dismissed as worthless by the AMA.

Echinacea is an herb that is extremely effective and holds multiple purposes. There are nine different species of Echinacea but the one most commonly used and referred to is the Echinacea purpurea. Many people take Echinacea every day to prevent colds, flu, and any other types of infections that might be running rapid at the time as Echinacea has been known for strengthening the immune system. Some people also use Echinacea for the treatment of acne and boils. The entire Echinacea plant including the roots are dried and made into teas, juices, and tonics.

While many swear by the power and strength of Echinacea there is no scientific backing that gives these claims any validity whatsoever. The Natives used to use Echinacea for many different things including the treatment of poisonous snake bites and insect bites. Back in the 1800's Echinacea played a very large part of United States medicine and then spread to Germany where they too used it for many medical purposes.

It was then used as an antibiotic and continued on until better antibiotics were made available. For years Echinacea sort of lost its pizzazz but more recently gained back its popularity. Many think the reason for that is because there is still no cure for the common cold.

There are many various parts of the Echinacea plant that are used to make medicine but most often it is the roots that are of the most value. Echinacea can be administered in many different ways such as in a tablets, capsules, juice, tea, extracts and tinctures. Some are made from the flower in full bloom and others are made from the root itself. Echinacea is also available in a topical solution or cream that many use for creams, lotions, mouthwashes, ointments, skin washes, and toothpastes. Further it is becoming quite common to add Echinacea to particular cosmetics as an anti-aging remedy but that claim has no validity at all as there is no relationship between anti-aging and Echinacea.

Echinacea is an extremely beneficial herb for helping the body rid itself of microbial infections. When combined with other herbs such as Yarrow and Bearberry it is said to work great combating cystitis however Echinacea has yet to be endorsed by the FDA for safety or effectiveness. Those who use Echinacea for the common cold swear by it and it is recommended that for the most effectiveness you should begin taking Echinacea when you notice the very first symptoms of a cold and then stay on it for three weeks and stop taking it for one week.

There are some who would be at risk if they took Echinacea such as people with multiple sclerosis, white blood cell disorders, collagen disorders, HIV/AIDS, autoimmune disorders, or tuberculosis. Heed caution also if you have any plant allergies; take other medications, or herbal remedies. Children should not take Echinacea, nor should pregnant women or nursing mothers.

Typically, side effects are not associated with echinacea supplementation. Mild side effects may include nausea or stomach discomfort, sore throat, headache, dizziness, body aches or fatigue. Orally-administered echnicea may cause temporary tingling or numbness along your tongue. Children in particular may be more likely to develop a skin rash as a side effect of echinacea treatment. People who are allergic to certain plants, such as marigolds, daisies, ragweed or chrysanthemums, may be at an increased risk of developing a severe allergic reaction upon exposure to echinacea,

# Eucalyptus

In 1777, on Cook's third expedition, the botanist David Nelson collected a eucalypt on Bruny Island, southern Tasmania. This specimen was taken to the British Museum in London, where it was named Eucalyptus. Eucalyptus is an aromatic herb that has properties that provide great relief as a decongestant and an expectorant. For centuries Vick's which is made as a Eucalyptus rub is applied to the back and chest of a person who has a common cold or any other respiratory distress. It is known to loosen the mucus in the chest so that it can be coughed up and expelled.

Eucalyptus also has some antibiotic association with it. Eucalyptus has both internal and external uses. Internally it is the leaves that are used for herbal teas that are able to assist people by acting as a diuretic, an anti-diabetic and also has some anti-tumor properties. The Eucalyptus oils are almost never used internally or ingested but on rare occasion a doctor might use a miniscule amount for nasal congestion, bronchial disease and other respiratory problems.

Externally, Eucalyptus is used as a vapor rub and while it is recommended that it be rubbed on the chest and back area it is also good for inhalation in such ways as steam vaporizers. Some even boil water and drop a teaspoon of vapor rub into it so an ill person can breathe in the fumes which will help to break up the congestion in the lungs. Quite often people have used the very same rub for sprains, bruises, and muscle aches and pains.

Never underestimate the power of Eucalyptus oil as it can be beneficial for many reasons. First it is a very powerful antiseptic, it is used to treat pyorrhea which is a gum disease. It is often used to treat burns too. One thing you can bank on is that insects do not like Eucalyptus so if you mix some with water and put it in a spray bottle you can be sure that bugs will stay away. A small drop on the tip of the tongue is said to take away nausea. Many people will soak a cloth in Eucalyptus and put them in their pantries or closets to fend off bugs and roaches. Another quick tip is a few sniffs of Eucalyptus is said to help someone who has fainted and when mixed with cinnamon is known to alleviate the symptoms of the flu.

Eucalyptus is also commonly used for aromatherapy too because when mixed with other oils it is extremely beneficial. The effects of Eucalyptus are stimulating and balancing and the scent is very woody. For the purposes of aromatherapy it blends well with Juniper, Lavender, and Marjoram. Eucalyptus when used in aromatherapy does the body good as it helps to relieve mental fatigue, improves mental clarity and alertness, sharpens the senses, refreshes and revives, stimulating, energizing.

It also has great effects on the body as it feels cooling; it relieves pain and sore muscles, breaks up congestion, and reduces inflammation. Eucalyptus incorporated with aromatherapy offers pure enjoyment. Inhaling the fragrance of Eucalyptus can reduce stress and lessen depression. It makes for an overall sense of better well-being. Eucalyptus is great for both bathing and also for massage oils.

Eucalyptus oil should be used moderately as it can cause skin irritation. It should not be used on children with five years of age or less. Eucalyptus supplementation is not advisable for children, pregnant women or women who are breastfeeding, older or chronically ill people. It should not be used by people suffering from low blood pressure, kidney problems, intestinal or biliary inflammation, stomach problems, or liver disorders. Eucalyptus may affect blood sugar levels. If taken in large amount, it acts as an irritant to the kidneys, by affecting respiration. The side effects of internal use of eucalyptus may include nausea, vomiting, and diarrhea. Overdoses of eucalyptus oil may cause life-threatening poisonings.

# Frankincense

Since farther back than anyone can remember Frankincense has been used for medicinal and religious purposes. Early Egyptians used Frankincense as part of their embalming process, the Greeks used it as an antidote to hemlock poisoning, and the Chinese used it for trading as well as for internal and external purposes. Today, Frankincense is used mostly for aroma therapeutics but many have also recognized it as an anti-inflammatory, antiseptic, and a diuretic. Some medical research has been done showing a relationship between the possibility of Frankincense and the treatment of osteoarthritis and may have some anti-cancer fighting agents.

Frankincense has also been shown to help with anxiety, disappointment, hysteria, emotional fatigue, nervousness, congestion, anti-inflammatory, immune deficiency, insomnia, asthma, bronchitis, emphysema, aphrodisiac, emollient, indigestion, carminative, antiseptic, expectorant, sedative, tonic, and anti-tumor.

Frankincense has been around since ancient times and is even mentioned in the Bible. The Jews offered up Frankincense in ceremonies. It seems that different regions use Frankincense for different reasons; the Chinese use Frankincense to treat leprosy, Egyptians used Frankincense to pain women's eyelids, hair remover, and perfume. The main contribution of Frankincense is for respiratory distress and although it was once taken internally but no longer is but now is rather used as more of incense and when it is infused with vapors it can help laryngitis.

Frankincense comes from a tree called the Boswellia Thurifera which can be found in Africa and Arabia. To get Frankincense, they split the trunk of the tree and allow the resin to harden before it is harvested. Frankincense is commonly used in the practice of Wicca which is a religion that practices witchcraft. They use Frankincense for perfumes and believe that it corresponds well with certain days such as Sundays and Wednesdays. What Wicca's call a solar spell is affiliated with Frankincense in the form of oil or herbs are used for spells and formulas that are related to solar issues.

According to the University of Colorado, boswellic acids derived from frankincense help to reduce cerebral edemas in patients suffering from brain tumors and resist leukemia cells. According to Colorado State Unviersity, boswellic acids exhibit potent anti-inflammatory properties. This can potentially help to reduce or negate the need for steroids--which have many negative side effects--commonly used to reduce inflammation in this medical condition.

These spells would be used for such purposes as physical energy, protection, success, and putting an end to specific legal issues. When you refer to Frankincense in the form of essential oils it is very expensive and is usually diluted with other oils or jojoba oil. These combinations are also used by the Wicca's when casting spells. Some people prefer to substitute Rosemary for Frankincense.

Ironically enough never forget that Frankincense was one of the beautiful gifts that were brought to baby Jesus on the night of his birth by one of the three wise men. This is also used to increase menstrual flow, to treat syphilis, for unsightly scars and stretch marks, and breast cysts. Further it is used to treat acne, boils, and skin infections as well. Frankincense is one herb that is not edible and is not known for use in any recipe contrary to those who believe that Frankincense is used in Indian cuisine. It is not known to be used in any cuisine at all but it is extremely helpful for the practice of aromatherapy.

# Ginkgo Biloba

Scientists thought that it had become extinct, but in 1691 the German Engelbert Kaempfer discovered the Ginkgo in Japan. The Ginkgo's had survived in China and there they were mainly found in monasteries in the mountains and in palace and temple gardens, where Buddhist monks cultivated the tree from about 1100 AD for its many good qualities.

Ginkgo-seeds were brought to Europe from Japan by Kaempfer in the early 1700's and in America later that century. Most of the earlier trees rose in Europe appear to have been males. The first recorded female tree was found near Geneva in 1814 of which scions were grafted on a male tree in the Botanic garden of Montpellier where the first perfect seed has grown. Now the tree grows in many countries all over the world as an ornamental tree.

Ginkgo is one of the oldest tree species that are alive and the leaves are one of the most studied leaves in clinical settings today. Ginkgo Biloba is an herbal form of medicine and in Europe and The United States is one of the biggest sellers. Many traditional medicines contain Ginkgo and are used for enhancing memory and to treat circulatory disorders. Scientific studies all support and validate these claims. Newer evidence shows that Ginkgo might very well be effective in treating decreased blood flow to the brain, especially in the elderly. There are two types of chemicals in Ginkgo leaves, flavonoids and terpenoids, which are thought to have very strong antioxidant properties resulting in aiding those who have Alzheimer's disease.

While the Ginkgo plant is still in tree form, it produces fruit that is not edible; inside of the fruit are seeds that are poisonous to humans. Most of the studies that are currently being conducted on Ginkgo are being done on the leaves of the Ginkgo (GBE). Although many components of the Ginkgo tree have been studied only two have been directly related to the big success of Ginkgo, as mentioned above. This is why Ginkgo is showing a much more structured relationship with treatment of Alzheimer's and Dementia. Because Ginkgo is so effective in improving blood flow to the brain and because of its antioxidant properties, the evidence that Ginkgo can help these patients is extremely promising.

It is suggested that Ginkgo truly can improve cognitive functions such as thinking, learning, and memory, improve activities of daily living and social behavior, and lessen the feelings of depression. Further studies are showing that the flavonoids can also help with retinal problems, people with circulatory problems in their legs, memory impairment, and tinnitus. Many doctors are recommending Ginkgo for treatment or discomfort associated with altitude sickness, asthma, depression, disorientation, headaches, high blood pressure, erectile dysfunction, and vertigo.

Ginkgo may also reduce the side effects of menopause, osteoporosis, and cardiovascular disease. The option of Ginkgo has a lot more appeal these days then the options of prescription medication which has unpleasant side effects. Children under the age of 12 should not use Ginkgo and in adults it usually takes about 4-6 weeks before you will see any significant results. There has been a relationship developing between Ginkgo as an anti-aging aid since it is such a powerful antioxidant that wards off the free radicals.

It is very common and becoming even more so for healthy people to include Ginkgo as an herbal supplement on a daily basis for better concentration and enhanced memory. People claim that in general they feel that Ginkgo reduces any mental fatigue that daily life has a tendency to bring forth. Many men are taking Ginkgo to improve impotence as well as increase fertility. The Chinese have used Ginkgo Biloba for many years and have found great success with it so it seems that they might be on to something here because this herbal remedy looks like it going to be around for a very long time.

If you are using anti-coagulant medication such as aspirin or warfarin you should avoid ginkgo biloba without consulting their physician. Those on monoamine oxidase inhibitors (MAOI) or who might be pregnant should also consult their physician before use. Side effects associated with ginkgo biloba are: increased risk of bleeding, gastrointestinal discomfort, nausea, vomiting, diarrhea, headaches, dizziness, and restlessness. If any side effects are experienced use of ginkgo biloba should be discontinued.

# Ginseng

Ginseng was discovered over 5000 years ago in the mountains of Manchuria, China. In the beginning it was used as food. By the third century China's demand for ginseng created international trade in the root allowing Korea to obtain Chinese silk and medicine in exchange for wild ginseng. By the 1900s, the demand for ginseng outstripped the available wild supply and Korea began the commercial cultivation of ginseng which continues to this day. The commercial harvesting of American ginseng began in Canada in 1716 after a Jesuit priest, working among the Iroquois, heard of the root so valued by the Chinese

Out of all of the herbal supplements on the market today, Ginseng is the most widely used. In earlier times Ginseng went by a different name, "man root." because the root resembled that of the shape of a man. To this day many people believe in the powers of Ginseng as they believe that it has healing and mystical powers. The Ancient Chinese thought that when a plant resembles a human body part that it would have a healing effect on that part of the body. In other words if a plant resembled a hand it would have the ability to heal the hands. But since Ginseng resembles the entire body it is thought that is can bring balance and well-being to the whole body.

Ginseng contains complex carbohydrates, is an anti-inflammatory, an anti-oxidant, and has anti-cancer elements. Notice today that many energy drinks contain Ginseng which is because it is known for creating energy, this was brought to the forefront by the Chinese but Americans have a different plan for Ginseng which is use it for mental lucidity and treating stress. There has been a growing relationship between Ginseng and its ability to strengthen physically as well as mentally and maintain good balance.

It was the Russians who actually made that discovery however the Asians have discovered that Ginseng helps mental improvement, eliminates anemia, and helps prevent diabetes, neurosis, coughs, asthma, and TB. Further they found that it can be very beneficial to the liver and can also reduce the effects significantly of a hangover.

There has been more recent research on Ginseng than on any other herbal supplement, ever. The concern is that many times when people purchase Ginseng at various stores it may have been over processed and therefore not as effective. The best way is to make sure that you are purchasing authentic Ginseng and in order to do that you may have to purchase the Ginseng root. Oddly enough, with all of the research and studies that have been conducted on Ginseng the FDA has yet to endorse it. It is known that people who suffer from high blood pressure, heart disease, bleeding or clotting disorders, or diabetes should not use Ginseng unless they speak with their physician first.

While it is true that Ginseng is most widely recognized as a medicinal herb it is also used quite frequently in teas and in cooking. Most people are aware of the infamous Ginseng tea but many are not aware that Ginseng is sliced and put into soups and often boiled and mashed, added to stir fry dishes, and added to boiling water when making rice. It is much more common for cooking in Chinese, Korean, and Asian foods.

Often Ginseng is used when cooking chicken and mushroom dishes. Many people also use it in desserts for some added zing. It is often used in soups, salads, and even jellies. It seems that most people who enjoy the benefits of Ginseng for cooking are vegetarians but it might be becoming more popular since people are now learning the true benefits of this very popular herb.

Medical researchers proved that Phytoestrogens in ginseng may accelerate the spread of breast cancer cells. Also, pesticide residuals have been found in Ginseng may also promote cancer. Headache, nervousness, agitation and trouble sleeping may occur.Ginseng may cause diarrhea, fast or irregular heartbeat, skin rash and unusual vaginal bleeding.

# Golden Seal

In prehistoric times, Native Americans, used goldenseal root for digestive disorders, including ulcers. They employed goldenseal root as a yellow dye, as an eye wash, and as a treatment for skin disorders. Iroquois found it beneficial for diarrhea, digestion, and whooping cough. Goldenseal became popular among Europeans, especially in the mid-nineteenth century when it was an official herbal remedy in the United States.

Golden Seal is a perennial herb that is part of the Buttercup family. Golden Seal is used for a lot of medicinal purposes in a variety of ways both topically as well as internally. There are actually quite a few ways to purchase Golden Seal, in a bulk powder, salve, tincture, or a tablet. Internally it is a great digestion aid and if gargled with it has been known to remove canker sores.

Golden Seal has been around since times of the European conquest of America but has remained very strong because even today it is used for anti-catarrhal, anti-inflammatory, antiseptic, astringent, bitter tonic, laxative, and muscular stimulants. Herbalists say that if you are trying to ease gastritis, colitis, duodenal ulcers, loss of appetite, and liver disease, Golden Seal is what you might want to look into which is available at all herbal supplement stores. Golden Seal is very bitter so it stimulates bile secretions, stimulates the appetite, and aids in digestion.

Golden Seal has been around since the mid-19th century but is now threatened because Golden Seal is one of the most over harvested herbs. It keeps getting harvested and harvested but never replaced. Golden Seal which also goes by the name Yellow Root is often combined with Echinacea and prepared for easing the symptoms of colds. It is the underground root of Golden Seal that is harvested and dried to make teas and both liquid and solid extracts that are then turned into bulk powder, capsules or tablets.

Scientists claim that there is no evidence to support the use of Golden Seal for any ailments or medical condition whatsoever because of the very small amount of berberine that Golden Seal contains. Regardless of scientific claims, Golden Seal is one of the most widely sold herbs on the market today.

Although a very controversial subject, many people believe that the reason that Golden Seal is standing solid ground in the marketplace is because it is used primarily for the purpose of masking positive drug screens for people who are required to take drug tests for work or through law enforcement agencies. Many claims there is no validity to this claim but still many people are buying it because a friend told them that it worked and for that matter it is promoted in High Times magazine for the sole purpose of covering bogus drug screens. The claim is that because THC which is the active ingredient in marijuana is fat soluble it stores itself in the kidneys and becomes water soluble. Two to three days prior to a drug screen, you get some Golden Seal, follow the directions and it's a guaranteed pass.

If Golden Seal is one of the most popular herbs on the market today then someone has to be keeping them in business and it is true that many people are turning to herbal remedies in an attempt to heal themselves naturally rather than load up with a bunch of prescriptions that have nasty side effects.

Serious adverse interactions may result from the concomitant ingestion of goldenseal supplements and drugs that are CYP2D6 and CYP3A4/5 substrates. Goldenseal supplements strongly inhibited cytochrome activities. The other side effects of goldenseal include skin, mouth, throat and gastric irritation. It may also cause nausea and diarrhea. Topical application of goldenseal or berberine may lead to photo-toxic reaction, after exposure to sunlight or artificial light sources emitting UVA.

# Gypsywort

Gypsywort is an herbal plant that but has no culinary purposes at all but rather is used for industrial and medicinal purposes. This plant originated in Europe and Northwest Asia. Gypsywort's most important properties come from the stem and the leaves. These were used for the astringents, sedatives, anxiety, tuberculosis, and heart palpitations. Industrially, Gypsywort was extremely beneficial in making a permanent black dye. Oddly enough that is how it got its name, the Gypsies were said to have stained their skin with this black dye like substance so they would resemble Africans or Egyptians while they were performing their "magic."

Gypsywort is also called Lycopus europaeus; it has no known hazards and usually grows near rivers, streams and ravines. You will likely find this plant from June to September but the seeds are the most ripe between August and October. A unique physical characteristic of this plant is that is has both male and female organs so it self-fertile, pollinated by insects and bees. In a survival situation, the root of the Gypsywort could be eaten raw or cooked.

The flowers of this plant are used for astringents and sedatives but also have an iodine property to it that is commonly used for hyperthyroidism. The entire plant has been known to slow and strengthen heart contractions, treat coughs and bleeding from the lungs, and excessive periods, and the leaves are great for cleaning wounds. Heart disturbances and nervousness can be eased by the use of Gypsywort. The part that is rendered for use is the flowering plant itself and the best time to gather these is June - September. It is a sedative, because it reduces the pulse rate in conditions involving an overactive thyroid gland by reducing the activity of iodine. It was once prescribed for hyperthyroidism and related disorders such as Basedow's disease.

Gypsywort can be purchased at your local herbal supplement store or ordered online and does have some outstanding benefits although not much culinary use. It is a very uncommon and not very often spoken about form of herb. Some use it with aromatherapy and a mixture of many other oils and fragrances. Bugleweed is very closely related to Gypsywort and for medicinal purposes the two are very often closely linked to each other.

The juice of the Bugleweed can also be used as a dye. The two could also be twins in the family of herbs. The rarity of this particular herb in underestimated and often undervalued. With the research that is being done each year on various herbs and their contribution to the medical field maybe one day people will hear more about this herb that remains quite a mystery to most.

Many of the other herbs that can provide similar benefits as the Gypsywort are becoming extinct because they are over harvested and over used so it could be extremely beneficial to utilize much rarer herbs that can often bring forth some of the same benefits as others. Gypsywort just might be one of the herbs that would fall into this category.

# Marjoram

The ancients believed that if marjoram grew on a grave it was a sign of the happiness of the departed spirit. Sometimes it was planted at gravesites to comfort the departed and ensure their eternal peace and happiness. In the middle Ages, bridal couples wore wreaths of marjoram to symbolize love, honor and happiness. It was commonly carried around in ladies posies and in sweet bags and sometimes strewn around the house as a deodorant. It was worn at weddings for happiness and added to food to nurture love. Marjoram was used in England at one time as an ingredient of snuff.

Marjoram is the dried leaves from an herbal plant called the Origanium hortensis. The name Marjoram is a Greek word that means "Joy of the Mountain." Ancient Greeks believed that if Marjoram grew on a grave that person would enjoy eternal happiness. The taste of Marjoram is a bit sweeter than that of Oregano. Many people believe that Marjoram is, in part, a species of Oregano. Marjoram is a pretty user friendly herb that is used quite traditionally in Italian, French, North African, Middle Eastern, and American cuisine. Marjoram compliments quite nicely sausages, various meats, fish, tomato sauces, salad dressings, breads, stuffing's, and salads.

Marjoram is a relative to the mint family. You get the most flavors from Marjoram if you use the fresh leaves rather than fried marjoram. One big difference between Oregano and Marjoram is while Oregano tends to prosper in taste the longer it simmers in a sauce or stew, marjoram is the opposite and should be added into the dish as late as possible. Although Marjoram is sweet and mild, it is also at the same time minty and has a hint of citrus. The biggest Marjoram exported in Egypt. Marjoram blends very well with Bay Leaves, pepper, and Juniper. While all vegetables can benefit from a hint of Marjoram, it seems to work best on adding and enhancing the flavor of cabbage and legumes. Marjoram tea is excellent for health and offers soothing effect. Marjoram tea is known to stimulate the sweat glands. Regular intake of marjoram tea during influenza can help ward off the flu virus and moisten stiff and dry skin.

Many people find a great benefit from Marjoram in aromatherapy oils. Marjoram is said to have a soothing and warming effect with a spicy and warm scent. This explains why it is so popular with those who enjoy the many benefits of aromatherapy. Many times for aromatherapy oils it will be mixed with lavender, bergamot, and cedar wood. Beyond the great world of aromatherapy Marjoram has many other beneficial uses too as it is used as an analgesic, antiseptic, antispasmodic, and as a diuretic. The many uses of Marjoram include treatment for anxiety, arthritis, bronchitis, bruises, colic, constipation, digestive problems, gas, insomnia, muscle aches and pain, PMS, Rheumatism, sinusitis, and sprains. The flavonoids in marjoram are supposedly good for cardiac health and are known to boost healthy arteries and heart by enhancing blood circulation and preventing cholesterol buildup.

Quite often people use Marjoram on a daily basis in various forms. Some prefer it as a tea which has been used throughout history for easing such ailments as hay fever, indigestion, sinus congestion, asthma, stomach upset, headache, dizziness, coughs, colds, and disorders associated with the nervous system. Some even use the tea as a mouthwash. One or two cups of marjoram tea per day have proven to be extremely therapeutic. Marjoram can be made into an ointment or salve by crushing the dried herbs into a paste, adding just a tiny bit of water. This is a common way to treat sprains and Rheumatism. Even still, some will mix the Marjoram into a paste and then into an oil to use for tooth pain or gum issues.

Pregnant women should keep away from this aromatic herb since over consumption of it can pose a slight risk of uterine contractions. Marjoram should not be ingested internally in a medicinal or herbal form during pregnancy but can be eaten as an herb that is added to food. As you can see, Marjoram is a very essential and beneficial herb that was used in ancient times and is commonly still used today.

# Oregano

Oregano has a very long history of use in folk lore. It has been used for culinary purposes, medicinal reasons, and was believed to hold magical properties as well. Much of its use in the past is still how it is used today. Ancient Greeks believed that oregano was a useful poison antidote and was used extensively both internally and externally as a fomentation to treat skin irritations and infections, dropsy, convulsions, and as an antidote for narcotic poisons. Traditional Chinese healers have also used oregano for generations to treat a variety of complaints. In Shakespearean times, oregano was used for just about anything.

If someone says Oregano, it is likely that you will think in terms of cuisine. You would be right as most people do think of Oregano is sauces and so forth. However, there are actual medicinal properties to Oregano as well. Oregano makes a luscious cup of savory tea that works well for gas, indigestion, bloating, coughs, urinary problems, bronchial problems, headaches, and swollen glands and to induce and regulate a woman's menstrual cycle. Others swear that is can cure fevers, diarrhea, vomiting, and same jaundice.

In the capsule form the leaves are dried and then crushed and placed into the empty capsule shell. Further, even others use the dried leaves by crushing them and adding just enough water to create a paste like substance and use it for a cream to apply for arthritis, itchy skin, sore muscles, and swelling. For a relaxing and soothing bath use Oregano leaves in the bath water. Finally, some people make Oregano oil and claim it helps rid toothaches.

In Jamaica people burn Oregano scented incense to ward off coughs and other respiratory distresses. Oregano has been used in ancient Greece and many other places across the globe where people have found a different use for Oregano besides cooking. Oregano is a perennial herb that is relative to the mint family and it is a very important culinary herb that is used in a lot of Greek and Italian cuisines. For cooking purposes it is the leaves that are used and while some like nothing but a fresh Oregano sprig, most will agree that the dried Oregano is much more flavorful.

Especially in Italian cooking you will notice a distinct relationship between the uses of Oregano in combination with Basil. The two always seem to create the perfect marriage especially in a tomato sauce. Oregano is also used on many vegetable dishes as well as a seasoning on various meats. The Greeks would never consider cooking with Oregano in their pantry. The famous Greek salad boasts its flavor of Oregano. No one could imagine eating a piece of pizza without a taste of Oregano added to it.

Oregano is commonly mistaken for Marjoram as the plants look very similar. Outside of the kitchen Marjoram and Oregano are best friends and do a lot together. The pair has quite plentiful properties in the areas of antioxidants and antibacterial. Together they are not only a great combination for flavoring food but also for preserving it too. Because both of their oils are perfumery they are placed in many different soaps and lotions. They are also used in combination for many potpourris and home décor.

There is no denying that Oregano has been around since ancient times both in and out of the kitchen. It had many medicinal properties then and it still does now. It was used in the kitchen and it is still used there now so those from ancient times started a tradition that is still followed to this day. Oregano's uniqueness is fully utilized in many different ways and will be for years to come.

Although beneficial, oregano is not an herb for anyone. Pregnant women and children should not use oregano. It contains emmenagogue properties, it can cause bleeding in pregnant women which may lead to miscarriage. Also, oregano oil is beneficial but should not be substituted for cooking oil to avoid irritation of the mucous membranes.

# Parsley

It is mentioned by the ancient Romans in the fourth century BC. Two types, one with dense crowded leaves the other with open, broader leaves are described. Pliny, in the first century AD writes that there would not be a salad or sauce served without parsley. The Ancient Greeks crowned winners of major sporting events with wreaths of parsley. One rumour had it that you could bring about the demise of an enemy by plucking a sprig of parsley while speaking his name.

When it comes to herbs, traditions have changed, varieties have increased, but through it all, Parsley has just stayed Parsley, flat or curly leaf, nothing major and no need for change. Use it as an herb or use it as a garnish, it does not matter people still love it. Often used fresh or dried, fresh is more popular and has very easy access when purchasing it or growing it. Storing it is simple, just wrap it is a damp paper towel and place it in a baggie and store it in the fridge. Parsley is used for all kinds of sauces and salads. Parsley can pretty much be added to anything and is used often to color pestos but it is very frequently used as a garnish.

Throughout history, parsley has been used for cooking as well as for medicinal purposes but has also been used for a lot more. Early Greeks used Parsley to make crowns for the Olympian winners. Hebrew tradition uses Parsley as part of Passover as a symbol of spring and rebirth. Parsley tracks all the way back to Hippocrates who used it for medicinal purposes for cure alls and as an antidote for poisons.

He also used it for ridding kidney and bladder stones. Many of these prior claims have been validated through modern science and it is true that Parsley is rich in vitamin A and C and is also shown to clear toxins from the body and reduces inflammation. Parsley has three times the amount of Vitamin C than oranges do!

Back in much earlier times, any ailments that was thought to be caused from a lack of Vitamin C was treated with Parsley such as for bad gums and loose teeth, for brightening what were considered dim eyes. The Greeks almost feared Parsley because it was associated with Archemorus, who too was an ancient Greek. Ancient tales tell that Archemorus was left as a baby on a parsley leaf by his nurse and was eaten by a serpent. For this reason the Greeks were terrified of Parsley which sounds kind of silly now but it took a while for them to get over that.

The parsley benefits even extend over to refreshing your breath after a meal. It kills bacteria for one thing. So it should really be eaten at the end of the meal for this purpose. It should also be eaten during meals to aid digestion. It is high in enzymes, which increases the body's ability to properly process not just in the digestive tract but also through the intestinal tract

Parsley was also used to regulate menstrual cycles because parsley contains apiol which mimics estrogen, the female sex hormone. Parsley was also used to ward off Malaria and is told to have been very successful in doing so and it aided with water retention as well. Although these are old wives tales as some might call them when you consider them for just a minute they really do make a lot of sense.

Some of these old remedies still are used in part today such as the use of Parsley for kidney stones, as a diuretic, for rheumatoid arthritis, as a stimulant, for menstrual regulation, to settle the stomach, and as an appetite stimulant. You can purchase Parsley juice at herbal stores and it can be very healthy for you although it might not taste the greatest it can be mixed with other juices to enhance the flavor. Dried Parsley really has the least amount of nutritional value to it.

But taking parsley oil isn't recommended for pregnant women because it may affect the fetus. This is one of parsley side effects. People with untreated kidney or gallbladder problem might also be adversely affected. It is highly recommended that you check with your doctor before taking any parsley essential oil.

# Rosemary

Rosemary was burnt at shrines in Ancient Greece to drive away evil spirits and illnesses. It was believed that a fresh twig beneath your pillow will away nightmares, or lay it under your bed for good night's sleep. A necklace made from rosemary preserves your youth and is said that it is also grown to attract elves. The Ancients were well acquainted with the shrub, which had a reputation for strengthening the memory. On this account it became the emblem of fidelity for lovers. In early times, Rosemary was freely cultivated in kitchen gardens and came to represent the dominant influence of the house mistress.

Rosemary was one of the cordial herbs used to flavour ale and wine. It was also used in Christmas decoration. Both in Spain and Italy, it has been considered a safeguard from witches and evil influences generally. The Sicilians believe that young fairies, taking the form of snakes, lie amongst the branches.

Rosemary is a relative to the mint family and the name is derived from its Latin origin to mean "dew of the sea." Rosemary is very common in Mediterranean cuisine and has somewhat of a bitter astringent taste to it. While that is true it compliments oily foods very nicely. A tisane can be made from the Rosemary leaves and that is also very popular when cooking.

First it is burned and then added to a BBQ to flavor various foods. Sage, unlike many other herbs has a high nutritional value to it and is rich in iron, calcium, and vitamin B-6 and is more nutritional in its dried form rather than fresh. Rosemary should be harvested just as you are going to use it because it truly loses its flavor once dried. Gardner's swear that if you plant some Rosemary plants in and around your garden, the Rosemary will fend off moths, beetles, and carrot flies.

Older Europeans loved Rosemary and believed that it improved memory and also used it as a symbol of remembrance and was often tossed into fresh graves before they were buried over. Traditionally it has been said that Rosemary, left untrimmed, would grow for thirty three years where it will reach the height of Christ when he was crucified. Many would also place sprigs of Rosemary underneath their pillows to ward off evil and nightmares. Often the wood that comes from the stems of the Rosemary plant was used to make musical instruments. Remember that people back then liked to utilize every piece of something as not to waste. Today, many wreaths are made from Rosemary as a symbol of remembrance.

Today, Rosemary is still used for many things besides cooking as it is in potpourris, air fresheners, shampoos, and cosmetics. There has also been scientific evidence that Rosemary works very well as a memory stimulant. Rosemary has also shown some cancer prevention properties in animals. But further Rosemary has shown a strong relationship in relaxing muscles, and to soothe stomach upset as well as menstrual cramps. The main thing to remember when using Rosemary for this purpose is that if you use too much it can actually cause a counter effect.

When made into a tea it is ingested for calming nerves and anxiety and as an antiseptic. Rosemary when used as a tea many people find to taste very good. Making the tea from Rosemary is quite simple actually, just pour boiling water over the leaves and steep for 10-15 minutes. A little sugar can be added by you should not add any cream. A few sprigs can be added to oils and vinegars to flavor the products which add a nice taste for cooking.

When used cosmetically it can lighten and tone human hair and when mixed with equal parts of shampoo it has been known to strengthen hair too. It also makes for a nice additive in hot bath water. Rosemary is still used quite commonly today however more so for cooking than anything else.

As with any supplemental herbs or medications, you should always consult with your health care provider when using rosemary. It is not recommended that you use rosemary in children under 18 years of age. Rosemary should not be taken by people with high blood pressure, ulcers, Crohn's disease, or ulcerative colitis. Rosemary oil can be toxic if ingested, and should never be taken orally. It may affect the blood's ability to clot, and could interfere with any blood-thinning drugs you are taking. Rosemary may interfere with the action of ACE inhibitors in high blood pressure medications like: Monopril, Vasotec, Zestril, Capoten or any other such medications. Rosemary may alter blood sugar levels and could interfere with any drugs taken to control diabetes.

# Sage

Sage also known as garden meadow; has a long tradition of culinary and medicinal use. Sage was once used to help preserve meat and over the past 2,000 years or so has been recommended by herbalists to treat just about every known condition, from snakebite to mental illness. In fact, in primitive times the French called the herb toute bonne, which means, "all is well". Modern research has shown that sage, while not a panacea, can help reduce excessive perspiration, digestive problems, sore throats, premenstrual cramps, and high blood sugar.

Sage is a relative to the mint family. It is common for Sage to be ground, whole or rubbed but is generally in more of a coarse grain. Sage is grown in the United States but is also grown in Albania and Dalmatia. Sage is a very popular herb in the United States and is used quite frequently for flavoring such things s sausage, pork, lamb, and other meats, salads, pickles, cheese, and stuffing. The smell of Sage is very aromatic and distinct.

Sage loves to hang around in the kitchen with Thyme, Rosemary, and Basil. They work very well together. Sage is normally one of the main herbs in stuffing for poultry but is often added to lamb and pork dishes as well. Sage is very strong and should be used sparingly as a little goes a long way. Sage, like many other herbs develops its full flavor the longer it cooks and withstands lengthy cooking times which might be why it is so good when used in the stuffing for the Thanksgiving turkey that cooks for about five hours.

If you grow your own Sage you will find that all you have to do is snip off the tops of the plant with scissors and add it right to your favorite recipe. Sage is still at its best when dried but if you prefer just simply place the fresh Sage leaves in a baggie in the freezer and pull them out as required.

Today, Sage has no medicinal purposes to speak of but back in a different time Sage was used regularly to cure snake bites and was also used to invigorate the body and cleanse the mind. In the middle ages it was quite common for people to make a Sage tea and drink it for ailments such as colds, fever, liver trouble, and epilepsy.

Although there is nothing to solidify these claims it is also said that a chewed Sage leaf applied to a sting or an insect bite will reduce the sting and bring down the swelling. Sage tea has been said to soothe a sore throat and also help in drying up a mother's breast milk and also reduces blood clots. Further it has been known to help with itching skin if it is added to hot bath water. Today, it is mainly the Native Indians who still rely on the herbal powers of Sage.

The word Sage means salvation from its Latin origin and is associated with longevity, immortality, and mental capacity. Sage never loses its fragrance even after being dried out so it is often added to potpourri and is also added to many soaps and perfumes. It has been used in insect repellents and has antibacterial properties which have helped it become a preservative for many things such as meats, fish, and condiments. Sage has a musky smoky flavor and works very nicely for cutting down some of the richness in many foods. It also goes great with almost any vegetable too. Sage is definitely an herb that most people almost always have in their pantry if they do any cooking at all.

Sage should also not be taken when you have a fever. Some individuals who take sage either as a seasoning or medicine could have an allergy to sage that can cause a reaction in their bodies. These reactions can include difficulty breathing, tightness in the throat or chest, chest pain, skin hives, a rash or itchy and swollen skin. Sage can cause cheilitis, stomatitis and dry mouth. Increases in blood pressure were also reported among some individuals who use Sage. Small amounts of sage consumed over a lengthy period of time can cause reactions in the body like increased heart rate and mental confusion. In extremely high amounts, sage can cause convulsions. For this reason, sage should only be taken of periods between           one           and           two           weeks. Sage extract should be taken carefully, since it contains high concentrations of thujone, and sage oil should never be taken straight dilute           it           in           water           before           consuming.

# Tarragon

Tarragon is a native of the Northern Hemisphere, particularly Eastern Europe, Eastern Asia, Northern America and Mexico. Artemisia, tarragon's genus, comes from the Greek goddess Artemis, known as Diana by the Romans, who was said to have given tarragon and other Artemisia's to Chiron, the centaur. History tells us that tarragon was not used by the ancients, but there were references to it in medieval writings as a pharmaceutical herb. It became popular in England in the 16th century, and came to the United States in the 19th century. It is believed to have originated in southern Russia and Siberia. The Tudor family brought it to England and planted it in their gardens there. True tarragon is unique in that it cannot be started from seed, but must be propagated by a cutting

Tarragon is a relative to the Sunflower family and there are two different breeds of Tarragon, Russian and French. However, when you go shopping and pick up some Tarragon for your pantry or a favorite recipe it is almost guaranteed that you have just selected the dried leaves of the Tarragon plant because that is what is most often used and sold for commercial purposes.

Tarragon has a somewhat bittersweet flavor to it, almost resembling anise with that hint of licorice flavor to it. Tarragon does not have a long history behind it like most of the other herbs as it was not brought into the Unites States until the 19th century. It does have some mention about being used in England much before that time though. Traditionally, Tarragon is used to flavor such things as vinegar, relishes, pickles, mustard, and other various sauces.

The word Tarragon is derived from the French word which means "little dragon." There are two beliefs about how this nickname came about; one is because back in early times it was thought that Tarragon had the ability to cure venomous snake bites. Other thought it got this name because of the distinct roots that the Tarragon plant has that quite clearly resemble that of a serpent.

However, sometime as early as the 13th century Tarragon became widely used for seasoning vegetables, inducing sleep, and as a breath freshener. Not until the 16th century did Tarragon become more widely known. The Tarragon that is sold in the US today is not true Tarragon but rather

Russian Tarragon which is not nearly the same. True Tarragon will be called French Tarragon and if you want to be sure that is what you are getting it is best to grow your own.

It is not recommended to use dried Tarragon because all of the active oils have been dried out. It is best to use fresh Tarragon which needs to be used rather sparingly because of its pungent taste. If you have grown the Tarragon yourself and have harvested it then put it in a Ziploc bag and stick it in the freezer. When it is time to use it there is no need to defrost it but remember that heat intensifies the flavor of Tarragon. If you have ever had Béarnaise Sauce, you should have recognized that Tarragon is the main ingredient in it.

Tarragon is used when preparing many sauces. In a pinch it has been said that a substitute could be chervil, a dash of fennel seed, or anise but the flavor will not be the same.

Many have claimed that Tarragon works well to induce appetite and the root of Tarragon was once used to cure toothaches. It is linked to medicinal uses for digestive aid and also for the prevention of heart disease. It can be used to induce menstruation and can be used as a sale substitute for people with high blood pressure. Further medicinal purposes include use for hyperactivity depression, and as an anti-bacterial aid for cuts and abrasions.

Tarragon is generally reported to have positive effects on health, with no side effects. However, some people may be allergic to the herb, and as such, refrain from its usage as herb, tea or essential oil.

# Thyme

The name comes from the Greek *thymos* meaning spirit or smoke. Properties attributed to thyme by the Greeks included the giving of valour and restoring vigour. The Romans also attributed these qualities, their soldiers bathing in it before battle to gain vigour, strength and courage. Later, in the Middle Ages, Knights would have a sprig of thyme embroidered on their scarves by their lady as a sign of their bravery. Its use is recorded yet earlier, by the Sumerians who used it as an antiseptic. The Egyptians used it their mummification brew. The sweet smell of thyme was enjoyed by the ancient Greeks and Romans to whom it was a compliment to "smell of thyme".

Thyme is a very popular and well known culinary herb. It is a very decorative plant while it is growing and is also very easy to grow as well but be prepared because bees just love Thyme. Many people use Thyme in stews, salads, meats, soups, and vegetables. Thyme is a very common household herb and is a member of the mint family. The plant is very aromatic and comes in many varieties. Thyme is a frequently used herb in many fish dishes. Oddly enough as much as honey bees love to suck the nectar from the Thyme plant is as much as other insects loathe it. Some people have been known to make a mist spray of Thyme and water and use it as a bug repellent.

Various forms of Thyme are available year round but many people prefer to grow their own. Nothing beats the smell and taste of fresh Thyme as long as you know to pick it just as the flowers appear. Once fresh Thyme is harvested it should be stored in either a plastic bag in the crisper or stood straight up in a glass of water on the shelf in the refrigerator for easy access.

The bad news, fresh Thyme does not have a very long shelf life, you will be lucky if it last a week. If you have selected fresh Thyme and decide to dry it then simply hang it upside down in a warm and dry atmosphere for about a week to ten days. Then you can crumble it into a powdery form and stored in a sealed dark container for no more than six months. You want to eliminate the stems as they have a tendency to have a woody taste to them.

Thyme has some medicinal purposes as well as an antiseptic, an expectorant, and deodorant properties as well. When combined with fatty meats Thyme has been known to aid in digestion too, especially with lamb, pork, and duck. Herbal medicine has used Thyme for various things such as extracts, teas, compresses, for baths, and for gargles. More modern medicine has chimed in and verified that Thyme just might strengthen the immune system.

Distilled Thyme oils have been used for the commercial use of antiseptics, toothpaste, mouthwash, gargle, hair conditioner, dandruff shampoo, potpourri, and insect repellant. It is also used in the production of certain expectorants that are prescribed for whooping cough and bronchitis. Thyme has also been used in part as an aphrodisiac and in aromatherapy oils as well.

If by some chance you are in the middle of cooking recipes that calls for Thyme and you find that you are out do not fret, it is said that you can use a pinch of oregano as a substitute if you have to. Thyme is very often used when cooking European cuisine but is essential for the correct preparation of French foods as it has that faint lemony taste to it. It has also been said that Thyme is one of the only herbs that a cook cannot over season with because the flavor is so mild. Thyme is a primary spice that everyone should have stocked in their pantry.

Thyme may be too strong for many people externally, so caution is advised. Some people have demonstrated sensitivity to the essential oil, so patch tests are appropriate. Thyme is often recommended by herbalists for the aid of children, however it should not be given to children unless as prescribed by a professional. Although it is safe to use thyme as a seasoning during pregnancy, high dosages should be avoided since it is a uterine stimulant.